Copyright Notice

Contents

Acknowledgments

As I near the conclusion of this brief booklet, I am overcome with gratitude for the people and forces who have led and supported me on my life-changing trip. Writing these words of thanks is a challenging task since gratitude is huge.

My heartfelt thanks go to my family, whose unwavering support and belief in my abilities have been my guiding lights. Your love and support have been my foundation, and I will be forever grateful for all of the sacrifices you have made to allow me to pursue my ambition.

I am thankful to my mentors and professors, whose knowledge and expertise paved the way for my studies. Your patient guidance, intellectual analysis, and enthusiasm for the art have influenced not just the content of this booklet, but also my professional growth. Bonds made on the training mat, the sharing of experiences, and the mutual pursuit of mastery have all been sources of inspiration and encouragement.

I'd want to thank the historical figures, prominent masters, and practitioners who have contributed to the Chinese martial arts culture. Your stories, lessons, and innovations have contributed depth and authenticity to the narrative in this booklet.

I'd want to thank my friends and colleagues for providing a sounding board for my ideas, sharing insights, and encouraging me. Your encouragement at difficult times and excitement in triumph have been a constant source of motivation.

I really hope that the pages of this booklet inspire, educate, and connect with the people who hold it. The words stated here have significance because you are interested in learning about Chinese martial arts.

As I thank the efforts of everyone who has played a role, big or little, in the preparation of this booklet, I am reminded that no undertaking is really alone. This work exhibits collaboration, teamwork, and shared passion. May the information, stories, and insights included within these pages stimulate your curiosity, heighten your appreciation, and aid you on your own path of discovery.

Best of health,

John Duval

Chapter 1

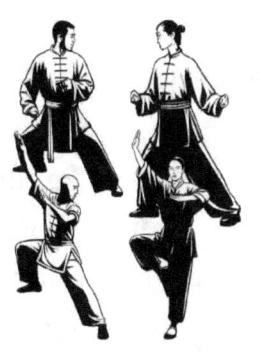

Introduction to Chinese Martial Arts

Kung Fu or Wushu, or Chinese martial arts, have a long and glorious history that is inextricably linked to China's cultural, social, and philosophical accomplishments. These martial arts provide a comprehensive approach to physical, mental, and spiritual well-being. By diving into their historical and cultural context, we learn about the origins and history of Chinese martial arts, as well as their enormous impact on Chinese culture.

The origins of Chinese martial arts are frequently obscured by myth and tradition, making it difficult to pinpoint their exact origins. According to mythology, ancient Chinese warriors studied animal and natural movements in order to acquire superior self-defense abilities. These discoveries are said to have led to the formation of the early forms of martial arts. Legends such as Bodhidharma allegedly introduced martial arts to the Shaolin Temple to emphasize the combination of spiritual and physical disciplines.

Chinese martial arts have strong philosophical origins in Confucianism, Taoism, and Buddhism. Martial arts principles of conduct and relationships reflect Confucian ideas of ethics, respect, and harmony. Taoism's focus on naturalness, harmony, and flow which is reflected in the flowing movements and energy growth techniques of many forms. In addition, the Buddhist emphasis on discipline, meditation, and compassion aligns to the mental and spiritual components of martial arts training.

Throughout Chinese history, several dynasties have made significant contributions to the creation and preservation of martial arts. During the Tang Dynasty, military books such as the "Ji Xiao Xin Shu" (New Book of Military Efficiency) were written, explaining war procedures and plans. Mongol and Chinese military strategies were merged during the Yuan Dynasty, resulting in new styles. Martial arts schools proliferated and styles and techniques were defined throughout the Ming and Qing eras.

China's large and diverse topography gave rise to a myriad of regional martial arts disciplines. Northern styles originated on the open plains, defined by explosive kicks and acrobatics, while Southern forms arose in the densely populated south, distinguished by close-range combat and strong strikes. These geographical variations were influenced by local customs, readily available training materials, and historical events.

Over millennia, Chinese martial arts have had an obvious impact on global culture. Impact of Chinese martial arts are considerable, from the spread of martial arts to adjacent countries to the establishment of martial arts schools all over the world. Movies, literature, and popular media have further pushed these abilities, associating them with notions of courage, persistence, and heroism.

As we explore the many varieties of Chinese martial arts, it is important to remember that their historical and cultural backdrop is a tapestry woven from a myriad of threads, each contributing to the rich and enduring history of these ancient traditions.

Chinese martial arts are built on a philosophy that encompasses principles about self-cultivation, ethics, and harmonious interaction with the world. This chapter delves into the philosophical foundations of Chinese martial arts practice, emphasizing key principles that guide practitioners on their road to personal growth and mastery.

Yin and Yang are key concepts in Chinese martial arts philosophy, representing the interplay of opposing forces and the dynamic balance that happens in all aspects of life. Practitioners attempt to bring these energies into balance in their movements and interactions with others. This idea influences techniques, footwork, and strategy by emphasizing the fluid transition between soft and hard, slow and fast, offensive and defensive.

Wu Wei is a Taoist concept that emphasizes effortless action achieved via natural flow and minimum opposition. Martial artists strive for "action without action," in which their movements become spontaneous and instinctual, allowing them to adapt to any situation successfully. This is shown by the smooth and economical movements of Tai Chi Chuan (Taiji Quan) and other internal martial arts.

Jing represents physical essence and endurance, Qi represents vital life force energy, and Shen represents intelligence and spirit. The capacity to balance and harmonize these components via breathing exercises, meditation, and focused attention increases a practitioner's overall well-being as well as martial proficiency. These three principles are the foundation of internal energy cultivation in Chinese martial arts.

The underlying premise of many Chinese martial arts disciplines is Qigong, which focuses on improving internal strength, flexibility, and balance via specific breathing exercises, postures, and meditation. This internal training enhances physical strength, technique, and mental clarity, all of which contribute to the overall competence and health of a practitioner.

Humility, respect, honesty, and compassion are examples of ethical ideals. Practitioners are encouraged to display these principles both within and outside of the training room, fostering a sense of belonging, mutual respect, and accountability.

To increase the effectiveness of their talents, martial artists develop precise intent when striking or defending against an opponent. This ideology emphasizes the connection of mind and body for the finest results.

The Five Elements philosophy (Wood, Fire, Earth, Metal, Water) is based on ancient Chinese cosmology and is used to describe martial arts strategies, tactics, and forms. Each element corresponds to diverse traits and movements that aid practitioners in adapting to different battle conditions.

He who accepts these philosophical concepts not only enhance their martial talents, but they also go on a journey of self-discovery, personal growth, and development. These principles serve as a guide, guiding practitioners to a deeper understanding of themselves, their art, and their place in the world. Keep these guiding ideals in mind while we explore the many schools of Chinese martial arts, since they are the substance that gives each technique and form life and significance.

Forms and techniques serve as the fundamental building blocks upon which the whole discipline is created in Chinese martial arts.

Forms, often known as "katas" or "taolu," arc choreographed movement patterns designed to embody the spirit of a martial art discipline. These forms comprise historical techniques, strategies, and thoughts that have been handed down through the ages. Martial artists maintain a direct relationship to the past by practicing forms that preserve their lineage's knowledge and heritage.

Forms are also a comprehensive exercises that engage several muscle groups, increase flexibility, and general physical conditioning. For the precise execution of techniques within forms, coordination, balance, and control are necessary, resulting in a heightened understanding of body mechanics and movement efficiency.

Technique repetition inside forms promotes muscle memory development, helping practitioners to execute techniques instinctively and properly in fighting situations. This muscle memory enhances reaction time and allows martial artists to focus on strategy and flexibility rather than specific mechanics.

Forms provide a controlled environment for practicing applications. Martial artists increase their ability to execute techniques effectively against hypothetical opponents by practicing striking, blocking, kicking, and actions within the framework of certain forms.

Learning and executing forms involve concentration and attentiveness. Practitioners must retain mental concentration in order to execute techniques successfully and maintain the flow of movement. This heightened awareness extends beyond training to promote mental clarity and presence in everyday life.

Forms also assist in the cultivation and circulation of internal energy (Qi) throughout the body. The coordinated breathwork, seamless transitions, and exact postures of forms assist in the channeling and harnessing of Qi, leading to improved health, vitality, and internal strength.

Forms are often used to monitor a practitioner's development and skill level. Martial artists advance by learning increasingly tougher forms that put their skills to the test and require mastery of previously taught approaches.

Forms and techniques convey the cultural history and identity of a martial art form and its practitioners. Form study and practice fosters a sense of belonging to a larger martial arts group as well as a shared cultural legacy. Remember how essential forms and techniques are in training the practitioners who bring these traditions to life as we travel through the many styles of Chinese martial arts.

Chapter 2

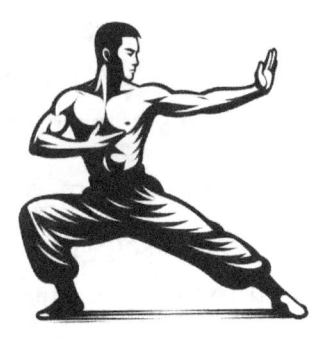

The History and Legends of the Shaolin Temple

Shaolin Temple is a legendary institution that gave birth to Shaolin Kung Fu, one of the most renowned and influential martial arts systems in history. It is located in the SongShen Mountain region of the Henan province of China. This chapter examines the origins, mythologies, and historical significance of the Shaolin Temple, tracing the evolution of its martial arts legacy and its profound influence on the world of combat and self-cultivation.

According to legend, the Indian Buddhist Bodhidharma (known as Damo in Chinese) arrived at the Shaolin Temple in the fifth century to spread Zen Buddhism. According to legend, Bodhidharma introduced a system of exercises and movements inspired by animals and nature, setting the groundwork for what would eventually become Shaolin Kung Fu.

The Shaolin Temple became a haven for travellers, scholars, and warriors, resulting in the exchange of various martial arts and combat techniques. Over time, the temple monks incorporated these diverse influences, refining and developing a comprehensive system of martial arts that emphasized both combat effectiveness and spiritual growth and Shaolin Kung Fu was created.

One of the most influential texts associated with Shaolin Kung Fu is the Yijin Jing (Classic of Muscle-Tendon Change), a treatise on physical conditioning and energy cultivation.

Numerous sources influenced the martial arts system of the Shaolin Temple, including indigenous Chinese combat techniques, Daoist principles of natural movement, and ancient battlefield tactics. This fusion of styles resulted in a formidable system of martial arts that emphasized powerful strikes, agility, and adaptability.

Shaolin Temple has played a pivotal role in the cultural and military history of China. Demonstrating the effectiveness of their martial arts, monks of the temple were frequently required to defend the temple's sacred grounds and neighboring communities from bandits and invaders. In addition, the temple served as a hub for cultural exchange, which contributed to the nationwide dissemination of information regarding Chinese martial arts.

Over the centuries, the Shaolin Temple has produced legendary martial artists whose exploits and stories have become a significant part of its legacy. From the exploits of the "Five Elders" to the tales of monastic warriors who defended the temple, these figures have come to symbolize valor, discipline, and military prowess.

As China's borders grew and trade routes flourished, the teachings and techniques of Shaolin Kung Fu spread to neighboring nations and beyond. The influence of the temple on martial arts is evident in the proliferation of martial arts disciplines in Asia and, consequently, their worldwide popularity.

The Shaolin Temple illustrates the enduring connection between physical training, spiritual growth, and cultural heritage. It provides a glimpse of where myth, history, and the pursuit of excellence intersect. As we delve into the fascinating world of Shaolin Kung Fu, we uncover the legacy of a temple that has left an indelible mark on the martial arts landscape and human history.

The development of the Shaolin martial arts system has been a fascinating journey spanning centuries, constituted of historical events, cultural influences, and devoted practitioners.

In its inception, the Shaolin martial arts system drew techniques from numerous sources, including indigenous Chinese martial arts, Daoist principles, and battlefield combat strategies. The temple monks diligently practiced and refined these techniques, gradually incorporating them into a system that emphasized both physical prowess and spiritual growth.

The monks of Shaolin developed forms (taolu) that embodied their martial expertise over time. These forms, which were inspired by animal movements, natural elements, and battlefield tactics, evolved into essential transmission vehicles for techniques, strategies, and fundamentals. Each form contained combat applications and specialized skills.

The constant adaptation of the Shaolin martial arts system to fluctuating conditions exemplifies the dynamic nature of martial evolution. As new challenges arose, practitioners refined techniques to address evolving combat scenarios, resulting in the emergence of sub-styles and specialized training methods within the larger system.

Internal and external martial arts were included in the evolution of the Shaolin system. Internal techniques emphasized the cultivation of internal energy (Qi) and the harmony of the internal systems of the body, whereas external techniques emphasized physical strength, speed, and explosive power. This duality motivated a strategy that balanced physical prowess with mental and spiritual growth.

Within the temple's walls, generations of devoted practitioners passed down the Shaolin martial arts system. The transmission of the system relied on a master-disciple relationship, with experienced monks passing on their knowledge and abilities to novices. Thus, distinct lineages and variants of the system emerged, each with its own emphasis and interpretation.

The Shaolin Temple's martial arts system had a profound impact on the cultural and social landscape of ancient China. Its emphasis on discipline, courage, and honor which inspired individuals from all walks of life to embrace its teachings, transcending social boundaries and fostering a sense of community and camaraderie.

As respect for the Shaolin system of martial arts developed, the temple became a hub for cultural exchange and dissemination of martial arts. The system's influence extended beyond the temple's walls, contributing to the development of other styles of martial arts and influencing the Chinese martial arts in general.

In modern times, the Shaolin martial arts system has continued to develop and adapt to contemporary contexts. Its influence on martial arts practitioners and enthusiasts has spread to every corner of the globe. Shaolin Kung Fu's incorporation into popular culture, film, and media has further solidified its status as a revered and iconic martial arts tradition.

The development of the Shaolin martial arts system is a testament to the tenacity of its practitioners and the profound impact it has had on the martial arts' history.

Shaolin Kung Fu, renowned for its dynamic movements, powerful strikes, and holistic approach, possesses a vast array of characteristics and techniques that make it a distinct and influential martial arts system.

Shaolin Kung Fu is characterized by its emphasis on explosive and dynamic movements. Practitioners execute techniques with speed and fluidity, transitioning from one movement to the next without pause. These movements allow for swift evasion, potent attacks, and the ability to adapt to changing combat situations.

Shaolin Kung Fu is well-known for its forms that imitate the movements and characteristics of diverse animals. These forms, which include the Tiger, Crane, Snake, and Dragon forms, offer practitioners a diversity of techniques and strategies based on the characteristics and strengths of each animal. For instance, the Tiger form emphasizes powerful strikes, whereas the Crane form emphasizes balance and accuracy.

Shaolin Kung Fu is comprised of a wide variety of hand and foot techniques, including jabs, strikes, kicks, and blocks. Techniques are executed with precision and intent, frequently incorporating circular or linear motions for optimal effectiveness. The combination of hand and foot techniques allows practitioners to maintain a diverse and extensive arsenal of combat skills.

Stances provide a solid foundation for both offense and defense in Shaolin Kung Fu. Practitioners are taught a variety of postures that enhance stability, mobility, and strength. Footwork techniques such as pivots, slides, and bounds enable practitioners to maintain optimal positioning and swiftly transition between attacks and defenses.

In addition to striking techniques, Shaolin Kung Fu also includes joint grips, throws, and grappling maneuvers. Using leverage and body mechanics, these techniques allow practitioners to control and immobilize opponents, thereby neutralizing or removing threats.

To enhance the practitioner's inner strength, endurance, and overall vitality, breathing exercises, meditation, and focused intent are utilized.

The Shaolin system of martial arts incorporates numerous traditional weapons, including staffs, spears, blades, and numerous polearms. Using the same principles as unarmed combat, weapon techniques are fluid, precise, and flexible.

Shaolin Kung Fu places a heavy emphasis on combat strategies and applications. Techniques are designed with utility in mind, allowing practitioners to respond effectively to a variety of attacks and opponents. The system's adaptability enables practitioners to adapt their techniques to differing ranges and conditions.

Shaolin Kung Fu is predicated on the cultivation of a strong mind-body connection. Practitioners learn to synchronize their movements with their respiration and mental concentration, enhancing their overall coordination, concentration, and awareness.

In addition to physical techniques, Shaolin Kung Fu teaches ethical values such as discipline, humility, and respect. Shaolin Kung Fu emphasizes personal development, self-cultivation, and the pursuit of inner harmony in addition to combat proficiency.

The defining characteristics and techniques of Shaolin Kung Fu provide a holistic and comprehensive martial arts approach that transcends physical combat.

There are numerous sub-styles of Shaolin Kung Fu, each with their own techniques, philosophies, and training methods. These sub-styles emerged as practitioners within the larger Shaolin tradition sought to specialize and refine their abilities over the centuries.

Tiger, Crane, Leopard, and Snake, followed by the Dragon. The characteristics of each animal are incorporated into the techniques, footwork, and strategies of every substyle.

Praying Mantis Style, also known as Tanglangquan, is characterized by its swift strikes, agile agility, and emphasis on capturing and commanding the movements of an opponent. This sub-style's techniques are influenced by the movements of the praying mantis and consist of swift and precise hand and limb movements.

The Northern Shaolin Style emphasizes, among other techniques, long-range strikes, acrobatic movements, and a diversity of postures. Due to its adaptability and complex forms, the Northern Shaolin Style is often associated with spectacular performances and demonstrations.

Unlike the Northern Shaolin Style, the Southern Shaolin Style emphasizes close-quarters combat, hand techniques, and practical self-defense applications. This substyle includes well-known systems including Wing Chun and Hung Gar.

Eagle Claw Style, also known as Ying Jow Pai, derives its name from the techniques of seizing and clutching. Practitioners employ intricate hand movements, joint locks, and pressure point attacks to subdue opponents. Additionally, Eagle Claw employs dynamic maneuvers and strikes as part of its arsenal of combat techniques.

The Drunkard Style, also known as Zui Quan, mimics the movements and actions of a drunk person. This sub-style uses erratic footwork and strikes to confuse and disorient opponents. It employs deceptive movements and unorthodox techniques for both offense and defense.

Hóuziquán, also known as Monkey Style, mimics the dexterous and malevolent movements of primates. Practitioners employ bounding, rolling, and other acrobatic techniques to avoid attacks and deliver erratic strikes. This sub-style's techniques emphasize adaptability and quick reflexes.

Bak Mei is characterized by its emphasis on close-range assaults and quick counterattacks. Combining destructive techniques with the cultivation of internal energy, it employs both external and internal principles. Bak Mei is renowned for its direct and effective method of combat.

These sub-styles emphasize the application of specialized conditioning techniques to develop exceptional physical capabilities. Iron Palm focuses on toughening the palms for powerful strikes, whereas Iron Shirt emphasizes conditioning the body to withstand impacts. These sub-styles are often associated with displays of physical prowess and perseverance.

Some sub-styles of Shaolin prioritize internal cultivation and energy labor, with Qigong, Tai Chi Chuan (Taijiquan), and Baguazhang being prominent examples. As integral components of martial arts mastery, these sub-styles delve thoroughly into the principles of internal energy, meditation, and mindfulness.

These well-known sub-styles of Shaolin Kung Fu illustrate the inventiveness and diversity of the martial arts tradition. Within the expansive framework of Shaolin Kung Fu, each sub-style offers a unique approach to combat, self-cultivation, and personal growth, demonstrating the countless opportunities for specialization and exploration. As we delve deeper into the complexities of these sub-styles, we discover the depth and complexity of the Shaolin legacy, which has been enriched by centuries of perseverance and innovation.

Chapter 3

Taijiquan (Tai Chi Chuan)

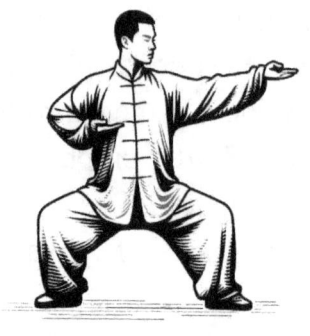 Tai Chi Chuan, commonly known as Tai Chi, is a profound martial art and holistic system that embodies the Yin-Yang philosophies. Tai Chi is renowned for its leisurely, meandering movements, with emphasis on internal energy cultivation, and on balance and harmony. This chapter explores the intricate relationship between Tai Chi Chuan and the Yin-Yang philosophy, examining how these principles influence the practice and philosophy of this fascinating martial art.

The concept of Yin and Yang, the fundamental duality that regulates the universe, is central to Tai Chi Chuan. Yin represents characteristics such as receptivity, yielding, and tenderness, whereas Yang embodies characteristics such as strength, firmness, and assertiveness. Tai Chi aims to harmonize and balance these opposing forces in both the practitioner's physical movements and his or her approach to life.

Tai Chi Chuan is frequently referred to as a moving meditation. Tai Chi forms' sluggish, deliberate movements to promote mindfulness, respiration, and an inner sense of peace. By coordinating respiration with movement, practitioners cultivate a state of tranquil awareness that promotes mental clarity and emotional balance.

The Tai Chi principles are a set of guidelines governing the execution of techniques and movements. These principles emphasize relaxation, energy submerging, proper body alignment, and Qi (vital energy) circulation. They guide practitioners in maintaining a connected, balanced, and efficient physical structure, thereby facilitating the flow of energy and optimizing health and combat effectiveness.

Tai Chi Chuan's central practice is the Tai Chi form, a choreographed series of movements. Each movement within the form incorporates the Yin and Yang principles, as well as other fundamental ideas such as opening and closing, expanding and contracting, and rooting and yielding. The practice of the form facilitates a thorough comprehension of these principles and their application.

Push Hands is a dynamic and interactive Tai Chi Chuan companion exercise that embodies the Yin and Yang principles. Practitioners engage in controlled pressing and yielding movements, learning to perceive and redirect the force of their opponent. Push Hands cultivates sensitivity, awareness, and the capacity to maintain balance under duress.

Tai Chi Chuan is also known for its graceful and delicate appearance, but it also has self-defense applications.

Tai Chi Chuan's inherent Yin-Yang philosophy extends to its profound health benefits. The practice promotes the equilibrium of Yin and Yang energies within the body, improves circulation, increases joint mobility, and alleviates tension. Regular Tai Chi practice promotes vitality, mental clarity, and overall health.

Tai Chi Chuan places a premium on the cultivation of Qi, or internal energy. Tai Chi forms' sluggish, deliberate movements promote the seamless circulation of Qi throughout the body's energy pathways (meridians), thereby enhancing health, vitality, and longevity.

Tai Chi Chuan emphasizes mind-body integration, nurturing a profound connection between physical movements and mental intention. This synergy enhances everyday awareness, concentration, and the cultivation of mindfulness.

Tai Chi Chuan is a voyage of self-discovery and development that reflects the ever-changing interplay of Yin and Yang. As practitioners delve deeper into the principles of Tai Chi, they discover the enduring wisdom embedded in its philosophy and the profound insights it provides into the nature of existence.

In the context of self-defense, the concept of sluggish and fluid movements in martial arts may appear paradoxical. Nonetheless, this strategy has been utilized to great effect in a number of martial arts systems, including Tai Chi Chuan and certain varieties of Shaolin Kung Fu.

Movements that are slow and fluent engage muscles, joints, and tendons in a deliberate and controlled manner. This form of exercise enhances flexibility, equilibrium, and posture. Practitioners cultivate heightened body awareness, ensuring that every movement is executed precisely and effectively.

Quick and forceful movements can contribute to exhaustion and loss of control in self-defense situations. Slow and fluid techniques conserve energy, enabling practitioners to maintain composure, implement precise techniques, and maintain concentration even during extended encounters.

Practitioners learn to synchronize their respiration, intention, and movement, thereby enhancing mental acuity and concentration. This heightened awareness is necessary for effectively perceiving and responding to hazards.

The principles underlying sluggish and fluent movements can be applied to a variety of combat situations. Practitioners can adjust their pace and intensity based on the circumstances, ensuring that their techniques are suitable for both self-defense and training.

The fluidity of sluggish movements permits practitioners to transition between techniques without interruption. This ability is indispensable for sustaining control and dominance in combat, as well as for redirecting the force of an opponent to their disadvantage.

Tai Chi Chuan, which has its origins in ancient Chinese philosophy and martial arts, has spawned a number of distinct styles, each with its own forms, principles, and training techniques.

Chen Style is the earliest of the main Tai Chi styles, with roots in Chen Village, Henan Province, and the Chen family. Chen Style, renowned for its explosive movements and combination of sluggish and rapid sequences, combines both forceful and gentle techniques. It consists of foundational forms such as Laojia (Old Frame) and Xiaojia (Small Frame), which highlight silk-reeling movements and intricate spiral patterns.

Yang Style, named for its progenitor Yang Luchan, is one of the most popular and well-known Tai Chi styles. It is accessible to people of varying ages and physical abilities due to its delicate and flowing movements. Yang Style emphasizes relaxation, balance, and mind-body integration. The well-known 24-Form and 108-Form forms are frequently practiced for health and relaxation.

Wu Style, was created by Wu Yuxiang and Wu Quanyou. It is distinguished by its compact and intricate movements, which emphasize precise positioning and the cultivation of nuanced energy. The Wu Style places a heavy emphasis on preserving a poised and centered body while performing movements.

Sun Style, created by Sun Lutang by combining elements of Xingyiquan, Baguazhang, and Tai Chi Chuan to create this distinctive form. Sun Style is characterized by nimble footwork, diminutive postures, and compact movements. Its emphasis on dexterity and adaptability makes it ideal for practitioners who wish to improve their mobility and joint health.

Wu Style, created by Wu Quanyou, was a student of Yang Luchan, and his son Wu Jianquan furthered the style's development. In Wu Style Tai Chi Chuan, balance, subtle variations in body positioning, and a compact frame are heavily emphasized. Its movements are marked by a sense of tranquility and fluidity.

In addition to these classical styles, contemporary Tai Chi practitioners have devised hybrid styles that draw inspiration from multiple traditional Tai Chi lineages. These styles frequently integrate elements from various schools, allowing practitioners to experiment with a wide variety of techniques and principles.

While many Tai Chi styles originated as martial arts, they are now extensively practiced for their health benefits as well. The sluggish and deliberate movements, in conjunction with focused respiration and mental concentration, contribute to tension reduction, flexibility, equilibrium, and general well-being.

Choosing a Tai Chi style is frequently a matter of personal preference, desired outcomes, and physical capabilities. Exploring various techniques and lineages enables practitioners to discover the subtleties and profundity of Tai Chi Chuan, thereby enriching their martial and holistic experiences.

Tai Chi Chuan practice provides numerous physical, mental, and emotional benefits that contribute to an overall sense of well-being. Tai Chi Chuan has captivated the attention of people worldwide due to its unique combination of delicate movements, mindfulness, and internal energy cultivation, which is rooted in ancient Chinese philosophy and martial arts. Some of the benefits of practicing Tai Chi Chuan is:

Flexibility and Joint Mobilization: The leisurely, fluid movements of Tai Chi Chuan improve flexibility and promote a full range of motion in the muscles and joints.

Muscular Strength and Endurance: Muscles are engaged when maintaining postures and performing controlled movements, resulting in increased muscular strength and endurance.

Balance and Coordination: The emphasis on stability and weight shifting in Tai Chi Chuan helps improve balance and coordination, thereby reducing the risk of falls, particularly in senior individuals.

Cardiovascular Health: Tai Chi Chuan practice promotes moderate aerobic activity, thereby promoting cardiac health and enhancing circulation.

Mindfulness and Meditation: Tai Chi Chuan's deliberate movements and focus on the breath induce a meditative state of mind, thereby reducing tension and promoting relaxation.

Cortisol Regulation: Regular Tai Chi Chuan practice has been shown to reduce cortisol levels, a stress hormone.

Mind-Body Integration: Tai Chi Chuan strengthens the connection between the mind and body, thereby promoting mental clarity, enhanced concentration, and heightened awareness.

Mindful Movement: Tai Chi Chuan practice necessitates focused attention on each movement, resulting in improved cognitive function and mindfulness.

Stress Management: The combination of relaxation, mindful movement, and respiration control assists in stress management and promotes emotional health.

Emotional Regulation: Through its meditative aspects, Tai Chi Chuan cultivates emotional awareness and regulation, thereby nurturing emotional resilience.

Tai Chi Chuan has been demonstrated to mitigate chronic pain conditions, such as arthritis, by increasing joint flexibility and decreasing muscle tension.

Injury Rehabilitation: Tai Chi Chuan's gentle movements can aid in injury rehabilitation by promoting progressive healing and strengthening.

Qi (Energy) Flow: Tai Chi Chuan's emphasis on cultivating internal energy increases the flow of Qi throughout the body, thereby promoting overall vitality and health.

Internal Strength: Regular Tai Chi Chuan practice helps develop internal strength, which supports the structural integrity of the body.

Body Consciousness: Practitioners increase their comprehension of body mechanics and posture, thereby enhancing their overall body consciousness and alignment.

Somatic Sensation: Tai Chi Chuan promotes enhanced somatic perception, which facilitates enhanced movement

Participating in Tai Chi courses promotes social interaction and a sense of community, thereby reducing feelings of isolation and fostering connections.

Graceful Aging: The delicate and low-impact nature of Tai Chi Chuan makes it appropriate for individuals of all ages, promoting healthy aging and preserving mobility.

Holistic Approach: The combination of Tai Chi Chuan's physical, mental, and emotional benefits contributes to an enhanced quality of life and increased longevity.

Tai Chi Chuan practice offers a profound journey of self-discovery, inner harmony, and well-being that transcends ordinary physical exercise.

Chapter 4

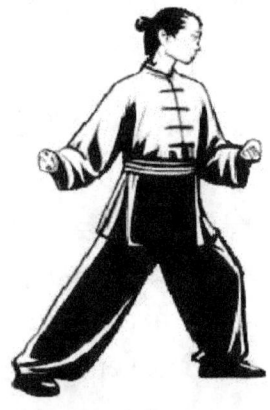

Wing Chun

Yim Wing Chun is the legendary figure whose name has become synonymous with the Wing Chun martial art form. Wing Chun is a unique and revered martial art known for its efficiency and directness. This chapter explores the captivating story of Yim Wing Chun, a tale that combines history, culture, and the indomitable spirit of a young woman who left a lasting legacy in the world of martial arts.

The setting of Yim Wing Chun's plot is southern China during the Qing Dynasty. During this period, pastoral villages frequently fell victim to bandits and oppressive forces. In this difficult environment, Yim Wing Chun's legend transpires, demonstrating her courage and determination.

A love tale that shaped Yim Wing Chun's destiny is central to her legend. According to popular accounts, Yim Wing Chun fell in love with a young man named Leung Bok Chau, who attempted to defend her from a local warlord who was determined to force her into marriage. Yim Wing Chun's voyage into martial arts was greatly influenced by the couple's closeness and shared desire for independence.

Yim Wing Chun is said to have found refuge at the nearby White Crane Temple in her pursuit of self-defense and empowerment, where she met the accomplished martial artist Ng Mui, a Buddhist nun. Ng Mui took Yim under her belt and taught her a self-defense system based on animal and natural movements.

Yim Wing Chun synthesized her martial arts knowledge with the principles of efficiency, simplicity, and directness under the teachings of Ng Mui. The ensuing martial art emphasized close-quarters combat, swift strikes, and simultaneous defense and offense. This system eventually became known as Wing Chun.

Yim Wing Chun's path was unorthodox in a society that frequently relegated women to subordinate positions. Her proficiency of martial arts defied conventional gender norms, demonstrating that skill and perseverance transcended societal expectations.

Through the martial art she helped to develop, Yim Wing Chun's legacy carries on. The effectiveness and utility of Wing Chun continue to captivate martial artists and practitioners worldwide. It has evolved and adapted over time, spreading to various regions of the world and inspiring generations of people pursuing self-defense, physical fitness, and personal development.

The influence and popularity of Wing Chun extends beyond the realm of martial arts. Its philosophy of reduction of motion, sensitivity, and adaptability resonates with people from all walks of life, and its techniques have been featured in films, literature, and contemporary culture.

The narrative of Yim Wing Chun functions as a metaphor for personal strength, resiliency, and the ability to surmount adversity. Her legacy inspires practitioners to pursue their passions, overcome their limitations, and embrace their inherent potential.

Yim Wing Chun's narrative embodies the spirit of devotion and self-discovery that characterizes the Wing Chun system. Practitioners pay homage to the legendary figure who defied convention and paved the way for future generations by engaging in the art's techniques, principles, and philosophy.

The story of Yim Wing Chun exemplifies the enduring capacity of martial arts to motivate and transform lives. As we investigate her extraordinary life, we disentangle the strands that connect history, culture, and the timeless pursuit of martial excellence in the form of Wing Chun.

The central principle of Wing Chun's combat philosophy is decreased motion. This principle stipulates that superfluous or ostentatious movements must be minimized, ensuring that every action serves a direct and efficient purpose. Wing Chun practitioners are trained to eradicate unnecessary movements and conserve energy, which enables them to execute techniques with speed and accuracy.

The centerline theory of Wing Chun is fundamental to its close-range combat strategy. The centerline, an imaginary line extending down the middle of the body, is a crucial offensive and defensive target. Wing Chun practitioners attempt to control and assault the opponent's centerline while defending their own. This tactic maximizes effectiveness by minimizing the distance between the attack and defense.

Wing Chun techniques are distinguished by their linear nature. Punches, strikes, and blocks follow direct trajectories along the centerline, which reduces movement and increases the speed and force of attacks. Using straight-line assaults, Wing Chun practitioners can deflect an opponent's attacks with quick, direct movements.

The simultaneous attack and defense strategy of Wing Chun permits practitioners to intercept and neutralize an opponent's attack while simultaneously launching a counterattack in a single, continuous motion. This concept corresponds with the principle of reduced motion, allowing Wing Chun practitioners to respond rapidly and effectively to shifting combat dynamics.

Wing Chun flourishes in close-quarters combat, as its techniques are optimized for arm's-length or closer engagements. The practitioner executes strikes, traps, and grappling techniques with minimal movement, exploiting an opponent's weaknesses while maintaining balance and position.

Wing Chun places a strong emphasis on sensitivity and entrapment, enabling practitioners to detect and control the movements of an opponent. This sensitivity to touch allows them to manipulate an opponent's extremities, throw off their equilibrium, and create opportunities for effective counterattacks.

The basic and effective technique of Wing Chun enables practitioners to maintain optimal positioning and control over the centerline. While executing techniques, footwork patterns emphasize stability, mobility, and the ability to maintain equilibrium.

Despite its emphasis on efficient movement and close-quarters combat, Wing Chun techniques are adaptable to a variety of circumstances. By developing a solid foundation in close-quarters techniques, practitioners can seamlessly transition to extended ranges if necessary.

The principles and techniques of Wing Chun have been demonstrated to be effective in real-world self-defense situations. It is well-suited for managing abrupt confrontations and ambush attacks due to its emphasis on direct, efficient movements.

The emphasis on reduced motion in Wing Chun encourages practitioners to be fully present and vigilant during combat. The practice cultivates mindfulness, enabling practitioners to perceive and respond with clarity and composure to an opponent's movements.

Wing Chun's reduction of motion and philosophy of close-range combat exemplify the art's practicality and effectiveness. Through the meticulous cultivation of efficient techniques, precise movements, and a profound understanding of combat dynamics, Wing Chun practitioners equip themselves with the confidence, agility, and skill to navigate the complexities of close-quarters engagements.

The Wooden Dummy is an iconic Wing Chun training aid. Its design imitates the shape and angles of a human opponent, allowing practitioners to practice techniques, strikes, and agility in a structured and controlled manner. The Wooden Dummy improves precision, timing, and sensitivity while providing striking and trapping techniques with a tangible target.

Chi Sao is an essential Wing Chun training method that cultivates tactile sensitivity, reflexes, and the ability to maintain contact with an opponent. Practitioners engage in continuous and controlled hand movements, learning to discern an opponent's intentions and respond with the appropriate techniques. Chi Sao improves adaptability and the ability to seamlessly transition between offense and defense.

Drills in Lap Sao emphasize grappling and capturing techniques, teaching students how to control an opponent's limbs and redirect their force. This form of training emphasizes close-quarters combat, allowing practitioners to neutralize an opponent's assaults and create openings for counterattacks.

Wing Chun's Biu Ji is a specialized technique that emphasizes explosive and penetrating blows. It is frequently employed as a last resort when in a compromised position. The objective of Biu Ji techniques is to incapacitate an opponent by targeting vulnerable areas such as pressure points and vital organs.

Chi Gerk trains leg techniques and footwork through controlled leg interactions, similar to Chi Sao for the arms. Practitioners gain balance, coordination, and the ability to maintain contact with an opponent's legs, enhancing their ability to control and defend against leg attacks.

Tao Lu, or Wing Chun forms, are choreographed sequences of movements that embody the art's principles and techniques. The Siu Nim Tao, Chum Kiu, and Biu Tze forms serve as repositories of fundamental techniques, advanced applications, and strategies for handling various combat situations.

Traditional Wing Chun weapons include the Butterfly Swords (Baat Jaam Dao) and the Long Pole (Luk Dim Boon Gwun). These weapons improve coordination, power generation, and combat strategy while illuminating the application of Wing Chun principles to external implements.

Single-sided techniques are utilized in Wing Chun, indicating that both limbs are used independently and interchangeably. This method maximizes efficacy by permitting practitioners to implement techniques with either hand, thereby eradicating the need to transition between dominant and supporting sides.

Wing Chun places a heavy emphasis on application in the real world. Practitioners engage in scenario-based training to simulate realistic self-defense scenarios, allowing them to test and refine their techniques under duress.

Wing Chun's distinctive training methods and techniques demonstrate its emphasis on combat effectiveness and adaptability. Through the intricate interplay of exercises, forms, and specialized techniques, Wing Chun practitioners develop a skill set that empowers them to navigate the complexities of close-quarters combat with efficiency and finesse.

Modern applications of Wing Chun continue to evolve as practitioners seek new methods to adapt its principles to modern challenges. Its enduring legacy is evidence of its usefulness and capacity to inspire generations of martial artists.

Chapter 5

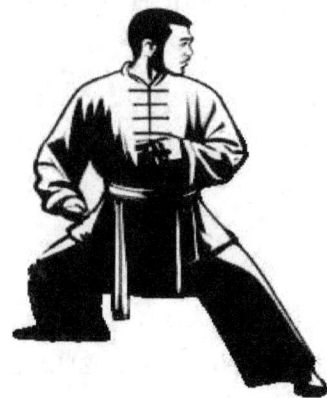

Baguazhang

Baguazhang, an enthralling Chinese martial art, is distinguished by its circular footwork and dynamic movements. This chapter explores the essence of Baguazhang, including the significance of its circular pacing and how its dynamic techniques create a synthesis of martial prowess, health cultivation, and philosophical profundity.

Circular footing is the defining characteristic of Baguazhang, setting it apart from many other martial arts. Practitioners move in fluid, continuous circles to create an intricate dance that maintains balance, fluidity, and a dynamic connection with the environment. Circular footing enables rapid direction changes, confusing opponents and facilitating seamless transitions between offense and defense.

Baguazhang's circular pacing exemplifies its fundamental principles, such as adaptability, non-linearity, and interconnectedness of movements. These principles reflect the cyclical nature of life and the natural world, nurturing a philosophy that embraces change and emphasizes harmony with one's environment.

Baguazhang is influenced by the I Ching's (Book of Changes) Eight Trigrams. Each trigram represents a distinct combination of Yin and Yang energy, which influences the movement's direction and essence. Circular footing follows the paths of the Eight Trigrams, imbuing the art with profound cosmological symbolism.

The dynamic movements of Baguazhang encompass a variety of techniques, including strikes, throws, joint locks, and evasive maneuvers. The circular footwork contributes to the dynamic nature of the art, allowing practitioners to generate power, redirect force, and maintain a constant state of movement that confuses opponents.

The circular footwork of Baguazhang facilitates the production and expression of spiraling energy, or Chansi Jing. This spiraling force increases the power and efficiency of techniques, allowing practitioners to strike, control, and manipulate an opponent's energy with minimal physical exertion.

Circular motion in Baguazhang has significant health advantages, enhancing cardiovascular health, joint mobility, and overall vitality. The continuous, undulating movements stimulate the passage of Qi (vital energy) throughout the body's meridians, thereby promoting health and balance.

Baguazhang's circular footwork promotes a meditative state of mind. Practitioners engage in meditative movement by synchronizing their respiration, intention, and movement. This aspect of meditation promotes mental clarity, emotional equilibrium, and heightened awareness.

Circular footing enables to elude assaults while positioning themselves for counterattacks. The emphasis on circular movement in the art produces a dynamic defensive strategy that confuses opponents and creates openings for strategic responses.

The circular footwork also extends to its weapon applications, enhancing the efficacy of the art with weapons such as the Bagua Broadsword, Deer Horn Knives, and the Bagua Staff. The agility complements the weapon techniques, allowing practitioners to implement intricate and fluent movements.

The circular footwork of Baguazhang reflects the inherent philosophy of change and adaptation in Chinese cosmology. It represents the cyclical nature of existence and encourages practitioners to embrace change, overcome obstacles, and flow with the ebb and flow of life.

The philosophy of the Eight Trigrams, which is profoundly ingrained in Chinese cosmology and philosophy, illuminates the path of Baguazhang as its guiding light.

The Eight Trigrams are a fundamental concept derived from the ancient Chinese prophecy text I Ching (Book of Changes). The Eight Trigrams are configurations of three lines that represent the dualities and interactions of Yin and Yang energy.

The philosophy of the Eight Trigrams emphasizes the cyclical nature of existence and the constant interaction of opposites which are fundamental principles in Baguazhang. Circular footwork and dynamic movements parallel the ever-changing interactions of Yin and Yang, allowing practitioners to respond fluidly to different combat situations.

The connection between Baguazhang and the Eight Trigrams philosophy provides practitioners with insights into the cosmic order and the governing principles of the universe. This association enhances their comprehension of the art's profound implications.

The philosophy of the Eight Trigrams provides Baguazhang practitioners with a philosophical framework for personal development and self-discovery. By synchronizing with the cyclical patterns of the Eight Trigrams, practitioners cultivate resilience, adaptability, and a profound connection with the natural world.

The influence of the philosophy of the Eight Trigrams secures the continuity and wealth of Baguazhang's legacy. As practitioners immerse themselves in the circular motion, dynamic movements, and underlying principles of the art, they become torchbearers of a timeless wisdom that bridges the divide between martial arts and spiritual insight.

The practice of palm adjustments and the cultivation of internal power are the essence of Baguazhang, providing practitioners with a transformative voyage that transcends physical technique.

Palm changes, a defining characteristic of Baguazhang, involve a series of circular and fluid hand movements that progress from one technique to the next. These alterations produce a continuous sequence of movements, nurturing adaptability, agility, and fluidity in combat.

Changes in the palm are imbued with profound symbolism, reflecting the interplay of Yin and Yang energies and the natural cycles. Each palm change embodies distinct characteristics, such as serenity, ferocity, or swiftness, reflecting the dynamic nature of the natural world.

Palm rotations serve as a means of balancing the body's internal energies. The spiraling and circular movements facilitate the harmonious flow of Qi (vital energy), enabling practitioners to access their internal reservoir of strength and vitality.

The adaptable techniques of Baguazhang extend to weapon defense. Circular footwork and dynamic movements allow practitioners to disarm or neutralize an armed attacker.

Even in high-stress situations, Baguazhang's emphasis on internal power development and meditative aspects cultivates a serene and focused mindset. This mental clarity facilitates effective decision-making and self-defense tactics.

Baguazhang's combat fluidity enables practitioners to effectively respond to threats with its circular footing, dynamic movements, and internal power development. Baguazhang practitioners furnish themselves with a potent system that enables them to navigate self-defense scenarios with confidence and skill by embodying the principles of adaptability, redirection, and versatility.

Chapter 6

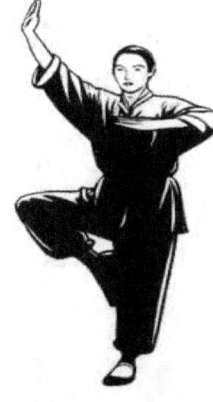

Xingyiquan

Xingyiquan, a formidable Chinese martial art, derives its power from the Five Elements' profound philosophy. This chapter explores the profound relationship between Xingyiquan and the Five Elements theory, revealing how this symbiotic relationship influences the techniques, movements, and underlying principles of the art.

The theory of the Five Elements, also known as Wu Xing, is a fundamental concept in Chinese cosmology and philosophy. It consists of the five elements of Wood, Fire, Earth, Metal, and Water, each of which represents distinct characteristics, movements, and interactions that govern the natural world.

Xingyiquan emphasizes the unification of Qi and Xing. The Five Elements theory provides a framework for comprehending how various energies manifest in the body's movements, enabling practitioners to harmonize internal strength with external techniques.

Each of the Five Elements corresponds to particular Xingyiquan movements, postures, and techniques. Practitioners imbue their techniques with the characteristics of Wood, Fire, Earth, Metal, or Water.

The Five Elements theory influences the stances and body mechanics of Xingyiquan. Practitioners assume positions that correspond to the characteristics of each element, thereby ensuring structural integrity, stability, and optimal power generation.

The Five Elements philosophy of Xingyiquan correlates with the energetic pathways, or meridians, of the body. Practitioners channel Qi along these conduits, thereby facilitating the efficient passage of energy and augmenting the effectiveness of their techniques.

Just as the Five Elements interact and influence one another in nature, Xingyiquan techniques fluidly and dynamically incorporate the attributes of various elements. Practitioners transition fluidly between elements, tailoring their techniques to the shifting combat dynamics.

The Five Elements theory informs the combat strategies and attributes of Xingyiquan. Each element possesses unique characteristics, such as the destructive power of Fire, the tenacity of Earth, and the precision of Metal, which practitioners strategically employ in combat situations.

Each distinct fist form in Xingyiquan is associated with a particular element. These forms embody the substance of the element's characteristics, guiding practitioners to cultivate particular qualities in their techniques.

The Five Elements theory extends to the internal alchemy of Xingyiquan. Practitioners endeavor to harmonize the energies of the Five Elements within themselves, nurturing equilibrium, vitality, and a profound connection to nature.

The incorporation of the Five Elements philosophy into Xingyiquan reflects the inherent philosophy of change and transformation in Chinese thought. Practitioners embrace the cyclical nature of the elements and alter their techniques and movements to flow in harmony with the fluctuations of life.

As we investigate the complex connection between Xingyiquan and the Five Elements theory, we discover a martial art that transcends physical technique and embodies the very essence of nature's patterns and dynamics.

Xingyiquan, a martial art renowned for its sheer force and focused precision, combines linear and explosive movements to create a formidable art which also involves direct and uncomplicated movements along a single path. These techniques maximize efficacy, enabling practitioners to rapidly close the gap with their opponent.

Explosive power is a distinguishing feature of Xingyiquan. The explosive movements of the art draw energy from the earth, channel it through the center of the body, and release it in an explosion of force. This explosive force generation is a defining characteristic of Xingyiquan's combat effectiveness.

The explosive movements are executed with strategic coordination. Practitioners utilize the element of surprise by discharging explosive force quickly and unexpectedly, thereby catching their opponents off guard. This incorporates both linear and explosive motions seamlessly. The linear approach amplifies the impact of strikes, throws, and joint locks by preparing the body for the explosive release of power.

Techniques involving explosives are refined for precise targeting. Practitioners concentrate their explosive power on particular targets, such as vital points or vulnerable areas, to maximize the efficacy of their blows.

Combining linear and explosive movements within combinations is a specialty of Xingyiquan. This synergy generates an unpredictable and dynamic flow of techniques, overwhelming opponents with a barrage of forceful actions.

The combination of linear and explosive movements in Xingyiquan amplifies the effectiveness of techniques while preserving their efficacy. Practitioners conserve energy by minimizing superfluous movements, ensuring that each explosive explosion has the greatest possible effect.

Imagination and visualization are involved in mental intent. Practitioners visualize the outcomes of their techniques vividly, which guides their movements and connects the physical and mental realms.

Xingyiquan practice fosters increased self-confidence and mental fortitude. Practitioners' confidence in their abilities is bolstered by their capacity to generate explosive force and respond effectively to threats.

The holistic training approach of Xingyiquan extends to life abilities. Its philosophy of adaptability, consciousness, and balanced energy provides a framework for decision-making and personal development.

Chapter 7

Tang Lang Quan - Northern Praying Mantis

Quick and agile strikes are hallmark characteristics of Northern Praying Mantis Kung Fu, a martial art celebrated for its lightning-fast techniques and dynamic movements.

Northern Praying Mantis emphasizes efficiency and precision in its strikes. Practitioners employ minimal and direct movements, ensuring that each strike is executed with the least amount of effort while maximizing impact.

Quick and agile strikes are characterized by explosive bursts of speed. Practitioners generate rapid acceleration in their techniques, catching opponents off guard and leaving little time for evasion.

The techniques often involve simultaneous attack and defense. Quick strikes seamlessly integrate with defensive manoeuvres, enabling practitioners to neutralize threats while minimizing vulnerability.

The art's quick and agile strikes excel in close-quarters combat. Practitioners deliver pinpoint accurate strikes to vital points, utilizing their agility to take advantage of an opponents' openings. Practitioners swiftly move in and out of range, maintaining optimal positioning for launching rapid attacks.

Central to the artistry of Northern Praying Mantis Kung Fu are its distinctive hand formations and trapping techniques, which exemplify the intricate and strategic nature of the style.

The Hooked Hand is a hallmark of Northern Praying Mantis. It resembles a mantis's front legs, allowing practitioners to trap and control an opponent's limbs. This hand formation is used for seizing, striking, and joint locking.

The Splitting Hand is characterized by the separation of the fingers into two distinct groups. This formation enables practitioners to simultaneously strike and manipulate an opponent's limbs, disrupting their balance and creating openings.

The Plucking Hand involves a swift and precise grabbing motion. It is utilized to seize an opponent's attacking limb, redirect their force, and set up counterattacks. This hand formation mimics the hooking action of a mantis's forelimbs.

The Crossing Hand creates a cross-like formation with the fingers. This technique is employed for controlling and trapping an opponent's arms, allowing for joint locks and strikes from advantageous angles.

The Triangle Hand forms a triangular shape with the fingers. This configuration is used to trap and immobilize an opponent's limb, granting practitioners control over the engagement.

The Hua Hand resembles the petals of a flower and is characterized by a circular, surrounding motion. It is utilized for trapping and deflecting an opponent's attacks, creating opportunities for swift counters.

Northern Praying Mantis excels in trapping an opponent's limbs and executing joint locks. Hand formations are intricately woven into these techniques, enabling practitioners to seize control and manipulate an opponent's joints.

Northern Praying Mantis traces its origins to Shandong Province, China. The region's martial heritage, historical events, and local traditions have played a pivotal role in shaping the foundational principles and techniques of the style.

The influence of Shaolin Kung Fu and internal martial arts can be observed in Northern Praying Mantis. Elements from these disciplines have been incorporated and adapted, enriching the style's techniques and philosophy.

Cultural reverence for nature and animal symbolism is reflected in Northern Praying Mantis's techniques. The art's mimicry of the praying mantis's movements embodies a cultural appreciation for the natural world.

Despite cultural and regional influences, Northern Praying Mantis Kung Fu remains deeply rooted in its traditional heritage. Practitioners honour the lineage and teachings while adapting to contemporary contexts.

Chapter 8

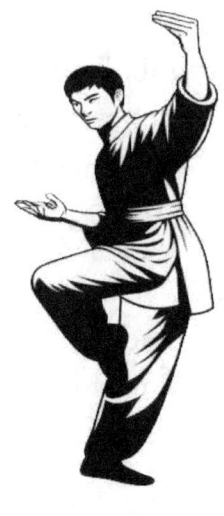

Bajiquan

Bajiquan, also known as "Eight Extreme Fist," is a martial art renowned for its brute strength, explosive techniques, and unrelenting aggression. This chapter examines the substance of Bajiquan, delving into how its distinctive approach to force and aggression has gained it a unique position among Chinese martial arts.

The name "Bajiquan" is derived from the Eight Extremes, which represent the eight cardinal directions and symbolize the art's expansive scope and versatility.

Bajiquan is distinguished by its explosive power production. Practitioners use their complete bodies to generate force, channeling it into techniques with unrivaled impact.

Aggression is a characteristic that defines Bajiquan. The techniques of the art emphasize a forward-focused strategy, overwhelming opponents with an unrelenting barrage of attacks. It emphasizes direct, minimalistic movements. Practitioners place a premium on effectiveness, executing techniques with concise and deliberate actions.

Bajiquan flourishes in close-quarters combat, targeting an opponent's vital points with brief, powerful blows. The brilliant techniques of the art are especially effective at close range. The strength derives from proper body mechanics and core engagement. Practitioners adept to timing and accuracy, exploiting openings and weaknesses in their opponents' defenses. Aggressive assaults are executed with pinpoint accuracy. It is also well-known for its direct assaults, but it also employs circular movements to increase power generation and disrupt an opponent's balance.

The strength and aggression of Bajiquan make it highly effective in actual combat situations. Its emphasis on overwhelming force is consistent with the requirement for prompt and decisive action.

Combative nature requires mental fortitude and conditioning. Practitioners cultivate a focused state of mind and emotional fortitude commensurate with the intensity of their techniques. Its reputation for short-range devastating assaults distinguishes Bajiquan as a martial art that excels in intense close combat.

In Bajiquan, close-range explosive assaults frequently entail simultaneous attack and defense. Practitioners intercept an opponent's movement while simultaneously initiating an explosive counterattack, resulting in an impregnable fusion of offense and defense.

Footwork is crucial to Bajiquan's close-range devastating assaults. Practitioners use expert agility to quickly close the distance and position themselves for maximum power production. Rapid and explosive disrupt opponents' synchronization and rhythm, creating openings for follow-up techniques or counterattacks.

Due to its emphasis on close-range devastating assaults, Bajiquan is particularly effective in realistic self-defense situations. The capacity of the art to impart rapid and overwhelming force correlates with the need for decisive action in close-quarters conflicts. Beyond devastating strikes, Bajiquan mastery also includes intricate combinations and joint locks that demonstrate the art's finesse and versatility.

Joint holds are utilized in Bajiquan to manipulate an opponent's joints and induce pain compliance and control. These locks are precisely executed, using leverage and angle to immobilize or submit an opponent.

Bajiquan's complex combinations and joint holds are designed to exploit an opponent's weaknesses. Practitioners evaluate the structure and movements of an opponent in order to employ joint restraints effectively.

Positioning and footwork are indispensable for performing complex combinations and joint locking. Practitioners employ clever footing to maintain optimal angles and control, thereby augmenting the efficacy of their techniques.

Chapter 9

Choi Li Fut

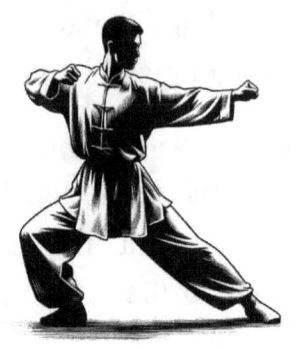

Choi Li Fut, an fascinating Chinese martial art renowned for its seamless fusion of Northern and Southern Kung Fu styles, occupies a unique niche within the domain of Chinese martial arts. This chapter explores how Choi Li Fut's synthesis of techniques, philosophy, and cultural influences produced a harmonious and dynamic martial tradition.

Choi Li Fut can be traced back to the legendary Chan Heung, who combined Northern and Southern Kung Fu styles to create a comprehensive and well-balanced system. His goal was to create a martial art that combined the best aspects of both traditions.

Choi Li Fut integrates Northern techniques, characterized by long-range kicks and agile agility, with Southern techniques, characterized by forceful strikes and intricate hand formations. This fusion produces a diverse repertoire.

The stances and footwork of Choi Li Fut represent the fusion of Northern and Southern influences. Practitioners utilize a combination of stable and flexible postures to facilitate rapid movement and dynamic transitions.

Choi Li Fut's hand formations and blows demonstrate the art's diversity. Techniques include quick punches, palm strikes, and intricate hand patterns based on Northern and Southern traditions. Circular and linear movements are harmonized in Choi Li Fut. Circular techniques seamlessly transition into linear strikes, allowing practitioners to transition between varying attack ranges and angles.

Internal principles, such as energy cultivation and body mechanics, are combined with external techniques in Choi Li Fut. This integration increases the effectiveness of the art while promoting holistic health. The art embodies the interaction of diverse traditions, which fosters a profound appreciation for Chinese martial arts.

The enduring legacy of Choi Li Fut resides in its capacity to evolve while honoring its foundational fusion. The art continues to attract practitioners in search of a comprehensive martial system that combines the Northern and Southern styles.

Choi Li Fut's dynamic movements are characterized by seamless technique transitions. Practitioners seamlessly transition from one stance to the next, producing a continuous flow of motion that puzzles their opponents. The flexible movement of the art enables practitioners to promptly maneuver and position themselves. The ability to control the tempo of a confrontation is enhanced by quick footing, which enables seamless changes in direction and range. Practitioners of Choi Li Fut are experts at combining diverse techniques in novel and unanticipated sequences. The adaptability of the art permits the inclusion of strikes, kicks, sweeps, and grappling techniques within the same combination.

Choi Li Fut demonstrates its versatility through its use of angular attacks. Practitioners can execute strikes from a variety of angles, exploiting the vulnerable areas and vulnerabilities of their opponents. The versatile hand formations contribute to the art's vitality. Practitioners utilize intricate hand patterns and strikes that transition fluidly between circular and linear movements.

The dynamic movements include strikes and takedowns, illustrating the art's adaptability in close combat situations. Practitioners are able to execute these techniques while maintaining motion fluidity.

The versatility of Choi Li Fut is equally evident in its defensive techniques. Practitioners are able to quickly transition from evasive maneuvers to counterattacks, neutralizing threats while maintaining a dynamic stance.

Choi Li Fut's reputation for adaptability extends to its mastery of both long- and close-range techniques, resulting in a martial art that excels in a variety of combat situations.

Front kicks, side kicks, and direct fists are among the kicks and blows included in long-range techniques. Close-range techniques include jabs, elbow and knee strikes.

Cultural exchange programs and international events provided Choi Li Fut practitioners with opportunities to share their knowledge and demonstrate the art's techniques, nurturing cross-cultural understanding.

Chapter 10

Traditional versus Contemporary Methods

The evolution and adaptation of Chinese martial arts have produced a dynamic interplay between traditional wisdom and contemporary innovation. This chapter explores how the intricate equilibrium between traditional and modern approaches in Chinese martial arts has influenced the past, present, and future of the martial arts.

The Chinese martial arts are steeped in tradition, with techniques, philosophies, and lineages that have been handed down from generation to generation. Traditional approaches emphasize cultural heritage and lineage preservation. Practitioners respect the teachings of previous instructors and strive to preserve the integrity and authenticity of their martial art.

The development of Chinese martial arts entails the incorporation of traditional philosophies into contemporary contexts. Practitioners reinterpret ancient knowledge in accordance with modern values and perspectives.

The refinement of techniques founded on scientific knowledge, biomechanics, and anatomy characterizes contemporary methods. Traditional methods are investigated and modified to optimize their efficacy and efficiency.

Modern martial artists investigate interdisciplinary integration by incorporating elements from other sports, fitness regimens, and scientific disciplines. This fusion enhances the practitioner's skill set and performance in general. Strength and conditioning, sports psychology, and data analysis are a few of the innovative training techniques utilized by contemporary training methods. These techniques improve physical fitness, mental fortitude, and strategic acuity.

Increasing cultural exchange and globalization benefit contemporary approaches. Chinese martial arts have acquired international recognition, resulting in the exchange of techniques and perspectives across cultures. Modernization has increased the accessibility of Chinese martial arts to a larger audience. The availability of online resources, instructional videos, and virtual training platforms allows practitioners to learn and practice regardless of their location. Practitioners achieve this equilibrium by preserving the essence of their art while adopting contemporary methods.

An examination of the development and adaptation of Chinese martial arts reveals a complex tapestry of tradition, innovation, and cultural exchange. The incorporation of traditional Chinese martial arts styles into modern contexts demonstrates their enduring relevance and adaptability.

Numerous traditional designs are favored for their health advantages. In contemporary contexts, these practices have been adapted to promote holistic wellness by enhancing physical fitness, mental clarity, and tension alleviation.

Traditional techniques frequently incorporate elements of mindfulness and meditation. These practices are incorporated into modern contexts in order to promote mindfulness, emotional well-being, and stress reduction. Adaptations are made to the practical self-defense aspects of traditional styles to address contemporary safety concerns. Individuals are empowered with effective self-defense skills by refining techniques for real-world situations.

Combat sports and mixed martial arts (MMA) practitioners value traditional techniques. The incorporation of Chinese martial arts enhances the athletes' skill set and adds an additional layer of strategy and variety to their learnings.

Curriculums at numerous educational institutions integrate traditional approaches. Schools, colleges, and community institutions offer martial arts programs that foster discipline, concentration, and character growth. The captivating techniques, philosophies, and stories of Chinese martial arts have left an indelible impression on various forms of entertainment and the arts as well as an permanent mark on the film industry. Films featuring legendary martial artists such as Bruce Lee, Jackie Chan, and Jet Li have exposed audiences around the world to the art's dynamic techniques and philosophies. Through dramas, series, and documentaries, Chinese martial arts have made their way onto television screens. These performances offer insights into the history, philosophy, and diverse forms of art that will always be cherished forever.

Chinese martial arts has also influenced fashion trends, with traditional attire, contemporary interpretations adorning catwalks and daily wear. Balance and harmony philosophy has also influenced wellness and lifestyle trends.

Music and dance performances have also been influenced, with choreography frequently integrating martial arts-inspired movements. These artistic expressions impart vitality, grace, and cultural resonance to performances.

Bruce Lee and other Chinese martial arts legends have become global cultural icons. Their contributions to the philosophy of martial arts and the entertainment industry have cemented their legacy.

The future of Chinese martial arts will be shaped by challenges and opportunities that will influence their evolution, preservation, and global recognition.

Chapter 11

Benefits for Children.

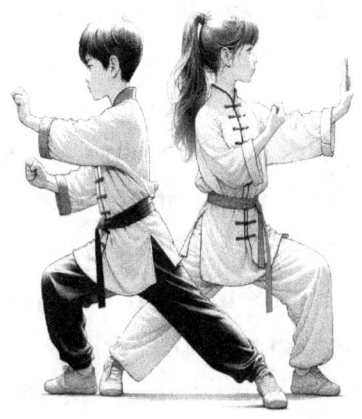

Chinese martial arts, such as Kung Fu and Tai Chi provide several advantages for both children and adults. These advantages extend to the physical, mental, and emotional aspects of health and well-being.

Chinese martial arts provide an unrivaled chance for youngsters to build core strength, which is essential for their stability and balance in martial arts techniques and good for lifetime physical health. These arts also improve flexibility, helping children to move more easily and lowering the chance of injury, both of which are important aspects of their general physical health. As a consequence of this intense exercise, their stamina and endurance improve, resulting in more energy and a healthier cardiovascular system. Martial arts practice also improves their balance and posture, which is vital during their formative years when their bodies are quickly expanding and changing.

Furthermore, the complicated motions required in martial arts training improve both fine and gross motor abilities, assisting in the development of exact coordination that may be used to other aspects of life such as sports and daily activities. Building muscle memory, which allows youngsters to do complicated actions with ease over time, is an important element of this training. This active participation in martial arts not only supports healthy physical development in a society increasingly geared toward inactive lifestyles for children, but it also instills lifetime fitness habits, making exercise a pleasurable and necessary part of their lives. This comprehensive approach to physical development via Chinese martial arts is a priceless instrument for instilling a healthy and active lifestyle in children from an early age.

Discipline and respect are fundamental aspects established in children via the practice of Chinese martial arts, and they have a significant impact on their personal development. This training goes beyond physical strength, instilling a strong sense of discipline that extends beyond the confines of the dojo or training hall. As they practice on a daily basis and seek to master different methods, children learn the importance of consistency, hard effort, and devotion. This discipline is about more than simply sticking to routines; it's about developing self-control, patience, and the capacity to endure physical and mental hurdles. Along with discipline, a major emphasis is placed on respect. Respect in martial arts is broad; it includes honoring the art, its history and culture, the teachers who pass on their expertise, and other practitioners who share the experience. Children learn to be courteous to others and to value their own and their peers' efforts and accomplishments. This regard goes beyond the martial arts environment, impacting how they engage with others in everyday life, developing healthy connections and a courteous attitude toward varied individuals and circumstances. Children acquire traits that form them into well-rounded persons, able to confront life's problems with elegance and integrity, as a result of the rigorous training and respect culture inherent in Chinese martial arts.

Children benefit greatly from the practice of Chinese martial arts because it develops an inner strength that is as vital as their physical ability. Children who participate in this ancient art form are constantly pushed to acquire new methods and push their limitations, which leads to a great feeling of accomplishment with each new skill achieved. This path of continual learning and conquering obstacles boosts their self-esteem as kids recognize their potential to attain objectives through perseverance and hard work. Furthermore, the encouraging atmosphere of martial arts lessons, where accomplishments are acknowledged and rewarded, helps greatly to their self-esteem.

Children grow to believe in their skills, and this belief spreads to other parts of their lives, whether it is in academics, social connections, or meeting new obstacles. Martial arts provide a feeling of empowerment that goes beyond physical strength to a profound conviction in one's skills and value. This idea is constantly reinforced as they advance, with each step ahead supporting their self-esteem and molding them into self-assured people. This transforming component of Chinese martial arts makes it a strong instrument in children's personal development, giving them the confidence and self-esteem they need to traverse the complexity of life with surety and grace.

Concentration and concentration are two fundamental characteristics cultivated via Chinese martial arts practice, and they have a significant influence on children's cognitive development. Children are taught to harness their mental energy in the regulated setting of martial arts training, concentrating intensely on the job at hand. Deep attention is required for learning the complicated motions and methods of martial arts, which require a degree of awareness that is both unusual and useful in today's fast-paced, distraction-filled society.

Children who learn to calm their thoughts and concentrate on their motions acquire an increased capacity to concentration that extends beyond the martial arts studio and into other aspects of their life, such as scholastic endeavors and everyday duties. As students learn to be more present in the moment and absorb information more efficiently, they enhance their memory recall and problem-solving abilities. Furthermore, the increased awareness and mindfulness gained from martial arts helps youngsters manage their emotions and behaviors, resulting in greater self-control and decision-making abilities. Thus, in Chinese martial arts, the emphasis on attention and focus is not only about physical prowess, but also about training a disciplined and alert mind, preparing youngsters for success in different aspects of their lives by strengthening their cognitive talents and mental resilience.

The Chinese martial arts training setting is a fertile field for developing social skills and collaboration in youngsters, and it plays an important part in their social development. Children who participate in martial arts lessons are exposed to a community that values teamwork and mutual respect. This community atmosphere helps students to engage with classmates from various backgrounds, therefore developing important social skills such as communication, empathy, and understanding. Teamwork is inherent in martial arts training, as students often team up for drills or sparring, learning to collaborate, anticipate each other's motions, and encourage one another in skill growth. This collaborative component teaches kids the concept of collaboration, demonstrating how working together may lead to greater accomplishments than working alone.

Furthermore, martial arts programs provide a regulated but supportive atmosphere in which children may make friendships and learn social niceties like as sharing space, taking turns, and applauding one other's triumphs. These encounters not only improve their capacity to work well as a team, but they also boost their confidence in social situations. The feeling of belonging and camaraderie that comes from participating in a martial arts class is priceless, giving youngsters with a supporting network and assisting them in developing into socially proficient persons. Chinese martial arts educate students with the tools they need to negotiate the complicated social landscapes of their future personal and professional life by strengthening these social skills and a feeling of collaboration.

Chinese martial arts are a great tool for stress alleviation and emotional well-being, which is particularly important in today's fast-paced, frequently stressful contemporary world in which children grow up. Martial arts provide a natural outlet for tension and anxiety, enabling youngsters to channel their energies and emotions in a controlled and healthy way. This physical exercise causes the body's natural mood boosters, endorphins, to be released, resulting in a sensation of relaxation and contentment. Aside from the physical components, several Chinese martial arts contain meditation and breathing practices that encourage mental tranquility and awareness. These activities teach youngsters how to regulate their emotions, exercise patience, and find inner calm. Regular participation in martial arts also fosters resilience, giving children the abilities they need to tackle difficulties and failures in a more balanced and collected manner. Furthermore, the discipline and attention necessary for martial arts training aid in the reduction of mental clutter and anxiety, resulting in increased mental clarity and concentration. Chinese martial arts provide children with a unique way to maintain emotional equilibrium and manage stress by providing a holistic approach to mental and emotional health, fostering a healthier, more balanced approach to life's challenges and contributing to their overall emotional and mental well-being.

Chinese martial arts practice introduces youngsters to the rich tapestry of Chinese culture, cultivating an appreciation that extends beyond the physical components of martial arts. Children who participate in these old rituals not only learn about diverse fighting tactics, but also about the historical and cultural importance behind them. This exposure to Chinese martial arts gives youngsters with a unique lens through which to examine and comprehend the deep concepts, traditions, and values ingrained in Chinese culture. Harmony, balance, and respect for nature, for example, are important to many Chinese martial arts and provide significant life lessons as well as a greater awareness of cultural variety and history. Furthermore, when youngsters learn about the beginnings and progression of various martial arts techniques, they acquire a feeling of respect and appreciation for the rich history and the individuals who have kept these traditions alive for years. This cultural education goes beyond the martial arts session, sparking interest and fostering a deeper research of Chinese culture, language, and arts. In today's globalized world, such cultural appreciation is critical because it fosters open-mindedness, tolerance, and a greater knowledge of the world's varied cultures. Children receive a well-rounded viewpoint by combining martial arts studies with cultural education, boosting their personal development and developing them into more culturally aware and courteous global citizens.

To summarize, the advantages of Chinese martial arts for children go well beyond the physical domain, providing a full developmental platform that transforms them into well-rounded persons. Children benefit significantly from the practice of these ancient arts in terms of physical fitness and coordination, creating a solid basis for a healthy and active lifestyle. Discipline and respect are instilled as basic principles in the disciplines, which are necessary for personal development and social interaction. Children gain confidence and self-esteem as they advance through their training, allowing them to confront life's problems with bravery and conviction. Furthermore, the attention and concentration necessary in martial arts training are crucial in improving cognitive capacities, which leads to improved academic achievement and problem-solving capabilities. Social skills and collaboration are organically developed in the collaborative and respectful setting of martial arts lessons, providing children with the tools they need to form healthy connections and work well with others. In today's fast-paced and sometimes stressful environment, the practice also gives a much-needed release for tension, encouraging emotional balance and well-being.

Above all, mastering Chinese martial arts allows youngsters to connect with and appreciate a rich cultural past, encouraging tolerance and open-mindedness. Each of these factors helps to children's overall development, training them not just as martial artists but also as balanced, disciplined, and culturally aware people ready to make their imprint in the world. Chinese martial arts' varied influence makes it an excellent exercise for children's physical, mental, and emotional development, developing them into healthy, confident, and culturally sensitive individuals.

Chapter 12

Masters and Prodigies

The history and legacy of Chinese martial arts can be traced to a lineage of exceptional instructors and legendary figures whose contributions influenced the art's development. This chapter explores the lives, accomplishments, and philosophies of some of the most renowned Chinese martial artists, demonstrating their indelible impact on the world of martial arts and beyond.

Da Mo (Bodhidharma):

Bodhidharma, regarded as the originator of Shaolin Kung Fu, is a legendary figure whose teachings at the Shaolin Temple established the foundation for the development and philosophy of the martial art.

Chen Yong Fa:

Chen Yong Fa is a modern martial artist who is a direct descendant of Chan Heung, the creator of the Choy Lee Fut Kung Fu style. Chen Yong Fa, the fifth-generation heir to this lineage, has been a key figure in the promotion and teaching of Choy Lee Fut across the globe.

Wong Fei-hung:

Wong Fei-hung, a renowned Master of Hung Gar, honored for his extraordinary combat abilities and dedication to preserving traditional Chinese martial arts during periods of cultural change.

Ip Man:

Bruce Lee popularized Ip Man's legacy as a maestro of Wing Chun, who was renowned for his Wing Chun expertise. Ip Man's contributions have been instrumental in Wing Chun's rise to international prominence.

Huo Yuanjia:

Huo Yuanjia, an accomplished martial artist and the founder of the Chin Woo Athletic Association, represents tenacity and integrity. His commitment to promoting Chinese martial arts contributed to their survival during a difficult period.

Li Xiao Long - Bruce Lee:

Bruce Lee is a pioneer in the martial arts and philosophy communities. His profound influence on martial arts cinema, his philosophy of self-improvement, and his innovative fusion of Eastern and Western ideologies have cemented his status as a cultural icon and an eternal source of inspiration.

Chen Wang Ting:

He was a member of the Chen Village Royal Guard in Wenxian County, Henan Province, in the 17th century. Chen Wangting is regarded as the inventor of the Chen Style, which is regarded as the oldest and parent form of the five traditional Taijiquan (Tai Chi) family forms. His creation of this martial art merged his military experiences, traditional Chinese medicinal beliefs, and prior martial arts training, resulting in a distinct style that combines slow, smooth moves with quick, explosive ones.

Wang Zi-Ping:

Wang Zi-Ping's contributions to Xingyiquan and Baguazhang have cemented his reputation as a proficient martial artist and protector of traditional Chinese martial arts.

Chen Long - Jackie Chan:

Jackie Chan personifies martial arts entertainment. His extraordinary physical skill, innovative choreography, and contagious charisma captivated audiences around the world, making him a celebrated figure whose legacy extends beyond film to philanthropy and cultural exchange.

Wang Xi'An:

Wang Xi'an, a well-respected figure in the world of martial arts, has devoted his entire existence to preserving and promoting Chen-style Tai Chi. Through his expertise, teachings, and dedication to sharing the art's genuine substance, he has become a beacon for those seeking to connect with the illustrious history of Chinese martial arts.

As we conclude our investigation into the diverse and captivating world of Chinese martial arts, we find ourselves immersed in a centuries-old tapestry of traditions, philosophies, and legacies. The voyage through the various styles, techniques, and stories has illuminated the profound impact of martial arts on the human experience, which is a dynamic combination of the physical, mental, and spiritual.

With their extensive history and diverse philosophies, Chinese martial arts offer more than just a collection of combat techniques. They facilitate personal development, self-discovery, and a deeper comprehension of the interdependence of the mind, body, and spirit. The principles of discipline, respect, and persistence that underlie these martial arts transcend the training mat and permeate all aspects of life.

As we consider the lives of legendary instructors who devoted themselves to the pursuit of martial excellence, we are reminded that their journeys involved more than merely physical endeavors. They exemplify the substance of what it means to be human: striving, learning, adjusting, and evolving. Through their stories, we see the resiliency of the human spirit and the grandeur within each of us.

We are invited to embrace the art of movement as a path to self-discovery, mindfulness, and holistic well-being as we embark on our individual journeys, whether as practitioners, enthusiasts, or inquisitive seekers. The lessons and insights garnered from masters and myths serve as guiding beacons, illuminating our path and inspiring us to cultivate our own discipline, fortitude, and knowledge.

As new generations of practitioners continue to contribute to its legacy and development, the exploration of Chinese martial arts is a never-ending journey. May the lessons and stories recounted in these pages serve as a source of inspiration, guidance, and reflection for all who wish to embark on this timeless journey of mastery, mindfulness, and the art of movement.

As we reflect on our investigation of Chinese martial arts, we are filled with respect and amazement at the immeasurable diversity and richness of this ancient tradition. The voyage through diverse styles, philosophies, and histories has revealed a captivating tapestry woven from centuries of devotion, innovation, and cultural influence.

The diversity of Chinese martial arts exemplifies the inexhaustible originality and creativity of human expression. From the sluggish, flowing movements of Tai Chi, which exemplify balance and harmony, to the explosive power and precision of Bajiquan, which exemplify controlled aggression, each style provides a distinct lens through which to comprehend the art of combat, self-discipline, and self-cultivation.

The underlying philosophy of Chinese martial arts transcends the physical techniques and invites us to explore the depths of our own being. Mind, body, and spirit integration is not merely a theory, but a lived experience that transforms practitioners into well-rounded individuals. Beyond the dojo, the emphasis on ethics, values, and personal development shapes how we navigate the complexities of life.

This gratitude is a tribute to the martial arts pioneers and visionaries who have dared to query the status quo, challenge conventional wisdom, and forge new paths. It is a commemoration of those who, with tradition as their foundation, have forged new styles, techniques, and philosophies that reflect the essence of the age.

Enter this universe with an open heart and an inquisitive mind. Embrace the difficulty of mastering new techniques, savor the thrill of pushing your limits, and revel in the company of other practitioners who share your enthusiasm. Similarly to how a river's currents flow in different directions, your voyage will lead you down unanticipated paths of growth and enlightenment.

May your journey be as profound as the art itself.

Best of health,

John Duval